YOUR VOICE, YOUR SUCCESS

EFFECTIVE GUIDELINES FOR YOGA TEACHERS AND EVERYONE WHO SPEAKS FOR A LIVING

TOMASZ GOETEL

ISBN: 9781521359389

Copyediting: Dale Jackson

Publisher: Tomasz Goetel / Save Me From Ruin Publishing No part of this publication may be reproduced, stored in a retrieval system, or transmitted in any form or by any means, electronic, mechanical, photocopying, recording, scanning, or otherwise, without the prior written permission of the Publisher. Requests to the Publisher for permission should be emailed to ubiktime@gmail.com

CONTENTS

CONTENTS

PART I

FIRST THINGS FIRST

THE BIG PICTURE

We need to be engaged and connected. We need to be right here and now, oozing enthusiasm and emotional intelligence. In teaching, training, and coaching we will not succeed without being present and engaged. Beware: we may be losing that ability since our society no longer upholds undistracted attention as the virtue it once was. One of the smartest ways to achieve presence and become engaged with others is to work on your voice.

As a teacher you are responsible for making sure that those you teach learn certain tasks and perform specific exercises. To be successful, you need a voice that commands attention—one that sounds strong, knowledgeable, competent, and compassionate. You want to teach your students with a firm approach and a soft heart. You want to feel that they trust you, rely on you, are happy to follow you, and eager to practice with you again. Your voice is a key factor in creating this reality.

Proficiency at chess, speaking a foreign language, or boxing all require conscious practice. Sounding great is a skill that can also be developed in this way, and because we are interacting with people all the time, we get to use our voice on a daily basis.

Of course, this can help you to gain more clients, more income, more success, and more satisfaction in your life. To make things happen, you need to listen to how you sound and then I will help you make the necessary changes.

Please keep in mind that merely reading this book is not enough to bring you maximum benefit. You would be short-changing yourself if you avoid all the exercises, even though they may feel odd at times. To be successful, you have to be willing to apply what you read in the book. When an exercise requires you to read a piece of text from a magazine out loud, that's what you must do. But not to worry. You will find this book to be easy to follow and easy to put into practice. Another good news: this book is rather small.

THE SMALL BOOK

You may have noticed that my book is shorter than other voice coaching books out there. You see, I have kept this book shorter as the things you need to know have been carefully selected so that we can focus on them. Also, by keeping the book short, I make it easier for you to complete reading it. I find that many voice books go too wide, too deep, and too long—people never seem to be able to finish reading them. The readers don't get to graduate, so to speak. So I made it my priority to be different.

Rest assured, you will encounter no big difficulties. You don't have to be super smart or talented to transform your own voice through this book. If you get lost, it's not your fault; it's because I might fail as a writer to keep you on the right path. In that case, please forgive me, and re-read the unclear section once more. I want to show you how easy it is to sound like a superstar—and when that happens, your professional life, and perhaps your personal life too, will immediately change for the better.

WHAT WE WILL COVER

You need a voice that commands attention. As a teacher you are responsible for making sure that people hear specific instructions and coordinate them into actions. Your voice should be strong, so that your students know you are a self-assured and knowledgeable person, but not too strong, so that they know you are a compassionate teacher. The goal is to teach with a firm, professional approach, but with a warm heart. We want to be partners in the learning process and have our students follow us, trust us, and become excited by all the beneficial possibilities we offer. The way you sound becomes a key factor in making all those good things happen. And let's not forget about making a good income and achieving the lifestyle you deserve—I want to change your voice into a money making machine.

I believe that once your voice sounds good, people are more likely to pay attention to you and your material, continue to listen rather than disconnect, believe you to be more interesting and competent, and overall, provide much better feedback—which is why I have written this book for professionals. It is not a course designed to educate you on all the anatomy and physiology of the human voice; the physics of how sound waves travel and how the ears receive them—those details are left out to focus on the practical things you need to know, to make you a more successful teacher.

All of us who are yoga teachers have one thing in common—we teach people. Whether one-on-one or a group activity, we speak to the people in front of us and rely on the successful outcome of those interactions to make a living. As a professional yoga teacher, I specialize in both private and group classes and spend a lot of time leading teacher training courses and workshops. We all communicate certain material to the person or group in front of us. They will be following what we say and do. As they observe, the instructions and demonstrations must be coordinated into action. The first keyword here is communication. We talk for a living.

As you begin to use the knowledge and techniques introduced in this book, you will soon realize that you may have underestimated the importance of having a wonderful voice.

On the other hand, you would not have bought this book had you not realized that having a great voice is the key to greater success in your line of work. Guess what: you are correct.

I'm going to coach you to achieve your own great success. But how do you define your professional success? I define mine as having more clients. (I call them students.) I find my success in the satisfaction of seeing how they improve. I like earning more money from my work—and perhaps being more popular, more sought after. Can you relate to this?

So we have the second keyword: success. Yes? What was the first keyword? Communication. These are the two main things we will concentrate on in this book. You will become a better communicator so that you can be more successful.

The best way to do this is to pretend it's just the two of us in a voice coaching session, no outside distractions and no one watching and listening, okay? Like a private, meaningful conversation. You can send me your questions by email, I will tell you more about this further in this book.

One way or another, the good news is that I'm a skilled and experienced teacher, so you're in safe hands. Plus, voice skills are easy to understand and improve. You will need a little practice. Let's check out the next chapter: how you can make sure you get the most out of this book—you will then be ready to get started.

HOW TO GET THE MOST BENEFIT FROM THIS BOOK

F ollow the specific lectures, examples, and exercises. Try to do everything I ask. If you get a little bit confused or aren't sure you understand something, feel free to go back over it again until you get it. There is no need to be in a hurry; I don't want you to rush and miss something you need to learn. Stay on the road laid out for you. Get through this book a little at a time, and you must reach the end in order to succeed. However, there are some things you may already be doing well, and other things which are particularly difficult for you. This was the case with my previous learners. If you want, you can read this book once as a whole, and then come back again to re-read the tricky parts.

This is important: learning is an active process; you learn by doing. Please, if you wish to master the knowledge you are acquiring through this book, do something about it. Not only when teaching yoga classes, but at every speaking opportunity, apply the voice principles described in the following chapters.

If you don't, you will forget them quickly. Knowledge is power, but only knowledge that is used changes the reality of our lives. You will probably find it difficult to apply the tonality principles all the time; I know because I wrote the damn book, and yet often I find it hard to apply everything I preach. So as we are going further into this book together, please keep in mind that you are not trying to improve your knowledge. You are trying to develop new habits.

Oh, I almost forgot: it's important that you have fun. I've been teaching yoga teachers for about 15 years now and always try to make sure our lessons are full of energy—even laughter. It's easier for us to learn and master new things when we're having fun. I hope you will enjoy your time with me.

As we go along, I will often ask you to record what you read and for this, you will need a book or magazine. You will also need to make voice recordings; you can use an app on your smartphone or computer, so please make sure you have everything ready.

ABOUT MY TEACHER

In 2004, when I attended Jimmy Barkan's yoga teacher training program in Florida, I was sure I knew what to expect: lots of yoga practice, lectures on anatomy and physiology, as well as several hours of teaching technique workshops. During the training, much to my surprise, I came to understand that teaching a yoga class is not about the subject itself, it's about teaching. And teaching is not about the material, but about the body and voice.

The "body and voice" training I got from Jimmy made me aware of how important it is (and how good it feels) to be funny, to be engaging, to be present, to listen. Jimmy Barkan's coaching created a supportive foundation for my future teaching career. Even more, it enabled me to become a better communicator in life: at work, the bank, restaurants, and in relationships. I realized that when the breath and voice are good—life is good.

Thank you for having this book in front of you. By the time

you get to the end, you will have a great voice, and you will love it. I will be so proud of you.

BREATHING AND SPEAKING

In a profound, metaphysical way, your breath is naturally linked to the length and quality of your thoughts. Simply put—breath and speech work like this: you breathe in, you speak out.

All of us breathe in different patterns. Individual patterns change depending on the circumstances, whether from the impact of an external influence or because of an internal condition, our breath changes with us.

As soon as you become interested in how you sound when you speak, you will begin to pay attention to how you breathe. Then, you begin to "think and feel" various words differently—in your head, in your heart, in your body—observing how others around you "think and feel" the words you speak. Words need to express feelings and thoughts, present material, and share ideas. Please understand that to be able to influence your students, not only will you need good words, but also a voice that results from the deep actions of your body, mind, and heart.

I have noticed that nowadays we tend to speak in shorter sentences with a broken rhythm, perhaps due to shorter breaths and a faster pace. We go through life in a flurry, so we rush our breath, and hurry as we speak. Or perhaps this happens because we want to explain a rather complex idea quickly. We don't want to waste our listener's time, right? We want to make a good impression. But this is counter-productive. We soon start to feel uncomfortable, gasping for air, clearing our throats, becoming red in the face, veins popping out from our forehead, eyebrows raised. Not a good look.

In this book, we will be working together to extend your breathing pattern (as a yoga practitioner you may be able to breathe well already). When your breath is extended, you will find that not only do you sound better, but you also think better, feel better, and emotionally express yourself better.

We will learn more about the breath a little later in the book.

Working with your voice is a journey of a thousand miles—beginning with a single word, and continuing always in the present moment, breath by breath, and word by word.

LANGUAGE = ENGLISH?

I f English is not your first language or not the language you use when you teach yoga classes—the information provided in this book will still work for you! In fact, I have applied the methods and exercises with non-English speakers before, and they work fine.

LANGUAGE = WORD CHOICES

If I am unwilling and unprepared to strive toward understanding and "owning" my words, I will be doing dull and mediocre work, lacking in creativity and satisfaction. I will be a robot instructor, a recording.

I commonly offer my yoga teacher trainees a piece of advice: learn to speak with easy, an open heart, and a clear mind.

"The truth needs to be experienced. Humans have the need to describe, to explain, to express what we perceive, but when we experience the truth, there are no words to describe it", said don Miguel Ruiz in his book The Voice of Knowledge. I look up to don Miguel, he is one of my teachers. There are no words to describe the truth? Oh, but don Miguel, we must try!

It is the mind that chooses the words, as language is the quality of the mind. The heart quality is also present within language, as the heart impacts the word choices, for instance, when we are choosing to say kind, supportive, or encouraging statements to our people in class.

Word choices play a significant role in our teaching. At the most basic level, it is good for us to stick to the plainest expressions when it comes to verbal cues for exercises. For example: when you want your people to lie down on their backs with feet toward the entrance, you tell them to "lie down on your back with feet toward the entrance." The ability to give clear, concise and well-chosen instructions is the mark of a master instructor —the students definitely appreciate it, I guarantee.

Various word choices carry different weight and energy. What words you choose and when you say them will directly inform people around you where you are from, how happy you are with your life, what your background is, how educated you are, what kind of sense of humor you have, and how intelligent you are. For instance, saying "don't slouch" and "find a way to sit straight" sound different to me, even though their technical objective is the same. They feel different. Keep in mind that many people, myself included, have a well-engraved dislike of being told what to do, and may be even more particular in their dislike of being told what not to do. Going further with the same example, they may be allergic to hearing such commonly used statements as "you should" and "you shouldn't." Any of those two, when repeated a few times in the same class, will give those students a skin rash. They will not like you!

We can also consider the difference in how we choose to present verbs. Let's use the verbs "take" and "turn" as examples. The most direct and commanding way would be to say the verb straight up: "Take a large step to the right and turn your foot out to the right." A less direct instruction could be worded like this: "Taking a large step to the right, turning your right foot out to the right." Want to be even less direct, and a bit more polite? How about this: "Find a way to take a large step to the right and

see if you can turn your foot out to the right." Yes, you're correct —that one doesn't work well, not for simple and essential actions. Here the straight-up version would work best: take, turn. If you prefer a softer approach because you're sick of being a military sergeant all the time in your yoga class, choose to mix up two versions, "Taking..., turn" or "Take..., turning..." But do avoid saying "turning... taking... inhaling... exhaling... stepping...," common among yoga teachers, where every verb has an -ing attached to it and nobody is ever told what to do.

The last, least direct choice "Find a way to..." can be useful for the more internal and less physical actions, such as when you are encouraging your people to breathe, rest, release, or digest. If that's the case, use expressions such as "Find a way to breathe gently," "Look for a feeling of calmness," or finally, "As you rest, allow the body to breathe and process information." I like the last line beginning with "As you (verb)..." and I use that often.

INTRODUCE YOURSELF AND ASK QUESTIONS

I would love you to introduce yourself, if you feel like it. Please write some comments or questions to me via email at tomaszgoe@protonmail.com. I always answer every question and do my best to resolve any difficulties you may have along the way.

PART II

THE BASICS

ALMOST EVERYONE HATES THE SOUND
OF THEIR VOICE

Now is the time for me to ask you to do something important. Record yourself and then listen to it. You will need to do it now, before we proceed further. Take a magazine, read from this book, or pretend that you are giving instructions to a group of people, but hit the record button on your smartphone and let it roll for a few minutes. When you've finished recording, play it back and listen to it. Ready? Again, you must do it now, before we go any further. So go ahead (then, come back after you have finished playing it back and listened to your voice).

What did you think? When people hear their own voice played back to them, they're usually shocked by what they hear.

Based on the sound of your voice, would you sign up to take your own yoga class? Would you pay yourself a higher rate? Would you hire yourself to teach that class on TV or online?

Most people would answer each of those questions with a big NO. They listened to a monotone, low-energy, flat-toned voice. Sadly, this may happen to be the voice that everyone else is listening to when you are teaching, day in, day out. It's the exact voice which is stopping you from achieving all the success you strive for in your work with your students.

Why haven't you done something about your voice before? If you've never thought seriously about how your voice sounds to others, please don't feel bad—that's normal. You simply didn't know there was anything wrong. We try to do well in life, but the sound coming out of our mouth is actually discouraging everyone around us from listening to what we have to say.

Or maybe you have tried voice training before but were unsuccessful? It's not your fault that the techniques you may have previously tried didn't work. As I mentioned earlier, I believe that many books and courses out there are too complicated, take too long to finish, or are unsuitable for a teacher or trainer. Never mind, okay? I know that this time, things will be different.

You must understand that you could be the smartest person around; you could be the most knowledgeable and experienced teacher around—all that doesn't matter if the people in front of you think you're not good. You need to always remember that people are listening and judging you based on the sound coming out of your mouth. There's no getting around it.

Fortunately, there is something we can do to turn that understanding to your advantage and make sure that everyone sees you at your absolute best at all times. This is so important for you to understand that I dedicate a separate chapter to it, coming next.

FIRST IMPRESSIONS

Whenever we encounter someone for the first time, in just one short moment, we form our impression of them. This process continues for the next few minutes, and there's more to it than deciding whether we like them or not. Based only on a quick look, we automatically make judgments about their age, upbringing, education, how much money they make, what their emotional state is, whether they would make a good friend or lover, or if they are a danger to us. You could say that this is superficial and unfair. Well perhaps it is—nevertheless, it's what we do. It's human nature to form an opinion about those we meet before we get to know them; there's no way around it. But wait, there's more!

Did you know that whenever a new person begins to speak to us for the first time, we do not necessarily listen to what they're actually saying but to what they sound like? Yep, that gives us even more information and... you guessed it, we make even more snap judgments about them.

First impressions tend to last. The fact that they are established quite quickly doesn't seem to matter—many first impressions are embedded and lasting, some may even be permanent. A person's general appearance and their tonality (what they sound like) count for a lot.

The bottom line is that when teaching yoga, people will judge you on the basis of their first impression. Understand that this is going to happen. The key is to discover a way for people to perceive you the way you want them to.

I will tell you a little story. I spent some time researching celebrities, and one of the things I wanted to know was what makes them so mega-successful compared to a normal person like me. First of all, I found that celebrities such as Rihanna, Brad Pitt, Eminem, or Anthony Robbins seem to be able to control the first impressions they make. Their appearance is not random and accidental, but chosen and self-regulated. Their tonality is controlled and often improved by training with a voice coach. For example, when in public and being interviewed on a talk show, they are in control of the following aspects:

1. Tonality (what they sound like when they speak).
2. Physiology (what happens to their face, hands, and the rest of the body).
3. Appearance (clothing and accessories).
4. What they are saying, the word choices they make.

All this is important for you to understand, become aware of, and perhaps make some improvements of your own. Your yoga students will always make judgments about you, beginning with their first impression.

Maybe I will need to write a separate book to cover the

important subject of first impressions. Would you be interested in reading it?

WHAT IS TONALITY?

I don't think that tonality (also known as vocal dynamics) is the primary reason behind the success of a yoga teacher but it must be very high on the list. Time and time again, while watching (and hearing) successful teachers whose rooms are always packed with people, I discover that they have a great voice to go with their performance. Not only do they consistently sound good, they are also able to adjust the sound of their voice at will. And they do it often! I hope that by now you have accepted the idea that how you sound can "make or break" your teaching success, even though there may be no such thing as a perfect voice.

Remember that if your voice is "high pitch" (high tone), while you're trying to get your students grounded in a posture, it's going to seem out of place. Your high pitch sound works against you, and although there's nothing wrong with it, when teaching yoga, the voice must direct energy and enhance the overall experience of those in the room, rather than working to undermine it.

Here's something you have probably never thought of: your voice could be destroying your teaching performance.

As discussed earlier, teaching a successful class depends on your ability to communicate. The actual science behind communication says:

* The specific words account for only 5% of any communication.

* 35% depends on your tonality—the way you sound when you speak.

* Over 50 or even 60% is determined by your physiology—what happens to your body when you speak (internally and externally).

The tonality of your voice is super important in all forms of communication, whether during a job interview, first date with an attractive stranger, or trying to sell your house to move to a bigger one with a swimming pool. When it comes to teaching yoga classes, having the right tonality is a huge advantage. First of all, to sound good, you must keep a good stance and breathe well. It's not what you say but how you sound that makes the difference. How do you improve it? Check your stance and breathe! The next chapter will cover those key areas for having a voice that sounds good.

THE STANCE AND BREATH

There are two points I want you to be aware of: stance and breath, and they must be put together to form a good habit. The two play a huge role in how you sound when you speak. Lungs exhale the air. The air passes over the vibrating vocal cords to produce sounds. For the exhaled air to pass over the vocal cords smoothly, the way has to be clear. If you crunch or slump your body, the passageways become restricted. Therefore, you must avoid dropping your head at all costs and never collapse the chest.

The Stance

Try this easy exercise:

1. Stand tall and upright so the air passage is open, and say, "Let's get started."

2. Stand and slump and say, "Let's get started."

Can you hear the difference? Try again: stand up taller, eyes forward, and say "Let's get started" once again. Can you hear (and feel) the difference this time?

Clearly, the position of the body has a fundamental effect on how words sound. When we slump, the words have a downward intonation that gives someone listening to us the impression that we are unhappy, disengaged, or bored! This may not be the case—in fact it probably isn't, but that is the message we send.

It's important that your stance provides an easy way for the air to get into your lungs. You need to look strong, comfortable, and competent. So as you will see, your stance makes a big difference to how you sound.

Let's try this one more time, with a little extra detail:

* Stand up straight, with your feet about a shoulder width apart.

* Roll your head around to ease any tension in your neck.

* Hold your head level with your chin, parallel to the ground, not tilted up or down.

* Raise your sternum, bring the shoulders back and down so that your chest is raised and open, which is what you want.

Watch out for:

* Slumping.

* Rounding your shoulders slightly forward.

* Beware of tension at the throat and upper chest (women).

* Beware of tension at the top of the stomach (men).

When you have a good stance and breathe correctly, your chest and shoulders do not move at all. That's a good thing. The only part of your body to change its position should be your stomach going in and out.

The Breath

We need to confirm that you're breathing well, and if not, we will make some adjustments. The foundation for working with the voice is to get it in the same rhythm as your body movements as you inhale and exhale. Breathing in a smooth and deep way is a wonderful thing for your body. The mind becomes calm and you find your center. The smooth, deep breath gives your voice power and consistency. I would like you to breathe in a calm and steady way, so that your voice sounds fabulous, enabling you to reach a whole new level in your teaching.

You are most likely skilled in this aspect already, but let's go through the basics, anyway:

* Stand in a relaxed way in front of the mirror.

* Take a deep inhale through your nose.

* Fill up your lungs as fully as possible then exhale the air slowly through the mouth. Take a mental snapshot of yourself in the mirror to remember how you felt inside.

When I ask a group of teacher trainees to take a deep breath, giving them the same instructions I just gave you, a lot of stuff happens. Shoulders pop up to the ears like elevators. Chests puff up like Popeye's forearms on spinach. But here and there, I will occasionally see a belly filling up—it's usually someone who has been told in the past that deep breathing involves filling up the lower abdomen. The exhale is sometimes forceful, with a push, as if they're trying to give birth. I can sometimes see the tension on their faces. Does this seem familiar to you? Did you notice your shoulders came up when you inhaled? Did you feel your chest puff up more? At the exhale, did you tighten your stomach to squeeze out all the air?

What you need to know is that there's no reward for putting all your effort and strength into getting it right. In fact, those things get in the way. Forcing and pushing your breath is exhausting. Solid, effective diaphragmatic breathing is just the opposite. It's easy and sustainable.

There is a simple three-step checklist:

Step One: Straight spine. Keep your spine straight, face and jaw relaxed, chin parallel to the floor and shoulders down and relaxed. Pay attention to alignment, this will help you eliminate much of the muscle tension that impedes good speech. An upright spine is important for projecting your voice. Whenever you are speaking in class, whether standing, kneeling down, or sitting—keep your bk straight. Make that a professional habit. You will breathe better and therefore project your voice better, but even more importantly, you will sound better.

Step Two: Inhale. You must inhale through the nose. The nasal passages contain nature's best air filters, which also condition the air. Importantly, they moisten the air coming into the voice box. Discover this for yourself: slowly, inhale deeply through your open mouth. Can you feel the throat drying up? Any person who is a "mouth breather" is going to be in trouble when speaking a lot for a living. Their voice strings will be strained, which eventually leads to loss of speech. So for all yoga teachers out there: when teaching, inhale strictly through the nose, okay? Oh, by the way, please don't worry that when inhaling deeply into your belly to speak, you will look fat. No one in your class will notice, I promise. You will actually sound better and therefore feel better.

I would like you to put your hand on your stomach, with your middle finger on your belly button. The other arm can remain alongside your body. All the action at the inhale should be taking place in the space between the lower ribs and just below your belly button. Let's keep your shoulders in a beautiful, open position (down, and back slightly); imagine that your stomach is a balloon, and as you inhale, it fills with air. Concentrate on filling the belly only. And when it's full, blow the air gently out through the mouth.

Step Three: Focus on the easy exhale. When you teach, you should only speak as long as you are exhaling. When the exhale is finished, you must inhale before you speak again. To help you achieve this, imagine the punctuations in your speech (commas, periods) and inhale right there when they happen. Practice it.

When you inhale, the belly needs to come out. When you exhale and speak, the belly needs to go back in without force.

There must be no tension at the top of the stomach. The upright spine must not collapse. The exhales must feel easy. You must let the air ride out unobstructed and free of stomach tension. When you learn to let your belly go in as the breath (and words) comes out, you are on your way to speaking with clarity, authority, and conviction. Airflow is a huge part of real teaching power!

THE FACE AND HANDS

E ven though you're reading a book on the subject of voice, I want to add some information for you about face and hands, because these are important.

The Face

I believe that one can hear someone smiling. Do you? When we smile, our voice is lighter and conveys fresh energy and happiness. When we look angry, the facial muscles affect our voice as well—the way we sound will be deeper and more stressed. Please remember that your facial expressions have an impact on your voice. During your class, your facial expression will unconsciously play a major role in how you sound and the communication process as a whole. You need to be more conscious of what the face is showing. As a general guideline, I recommend you find a way to achieve a "neutral expression": not blank, but a "mini–smile."

The Hands

Allowing your hands to drop with arms at your side when teaching a class may be a comfortable habit for you. Perhaps it takes less energy and makes you feel more relaxed about the job. Unfortunately, dropping your arms may have unwanted consequences—you will look and sound low and boring to the people in front of you.

Please remember not to make that mistake and get in the habit of checking yourself: when you drop your arms and stand still, the voice also loses its power in a big way. This boring tone usually drops even further at the end of each instruction, which results in a downward intonation that can easily put your people to sleep or into a depressed state if the voice is quiet. Alternatively, you may be perceived as aggressive and controlling if your voice is too loud.

According to some of the insights I've gained while looking into the latest findings on the science of body language and human behavior, there are only two good reasons for dropping the arms: to walk or stand. That's why many instructors who would stand in one place with their arms down, eventually begin pacing back and forth. This appears shifty, unnatural, and creates a bad impression. The brain tells us that with our arms at our sides we should be moving, especially when people are looking at us. But when we stand still, arms hanging down, the body takes it as a signal to rest. That may be the main reason why you and your group start to get sleepy in class: if you are standing still with your arms hanging down as you speak, your heart rate, blood pressure, and energy level will decline pretty fast. The voice follows suit and drops in tone— things can only go downhill from there.

You will get better results if you keep your hands at the level of your belly most of the time, and at the chest level some of the time. Make all your gestures there.

When your intention is to have a group of people place their confidence in you, place your hands at the level of your belly and perform open gestures from there. This will affect how you look and the sound of your voice in a profound, trustworthy, positive way. When the hands make gestures at belly level, an energized but balanced, calm and confident effect is felt both by you and the people in front of you. Having your hands level with your belly not only affects your body language, but also the way you sound, which in turn influences the way the group receives you and your material. This idea of gesturing within your belly area is very effective—it will positively influence the way you sound—and that's without hours of vocal training with expensive coaches or courses.

When you shift your hands up to chest height, you will notice another difference. By making gestures at a little over sternum level, your breathing rate, and sometimes even your heart rate, speeds up. You will be breathing more into your chest rather than the belly. When you are gesturing with your hands at chest level, you're making people think that there is more to come: it creates a bit of suspense, which helps in getting people to listen to you. If your hands come up to your chest when you gesture or speak, especially in contrast to the low energy and depressed way of speaking with dropped arms, or the "trustworthy" balance of keeping your hands in the belly area—people will notice a great difference. It will be like receiving a call to action! Gestures at chest level. Keep this idea in mind, powerful yet simple stuff.

PART III

HOW TO SOUND BETTER

VOLUME

You need a lot of volume (loudness) so that the students can hear you. There's nothing that annoys, bores, and turns people off more than being unable to hear you.

You're Too Quiet

Your volume needs to show everyone that you mean business. Please don't think that you are shouting or appearing angry. We will add melody to your voice later in the book. When you have more melody, people will think of you as a competent, passionate, and compassionate helper.

In the meantime, you must learn how to speak up! This is difficult for many of us, whether as a result of our upbringing or cultural standards—we may think it impolite to speak loudly. Or perhaps we are simply not used to it?

Not long ago, I was coaching a yoga teacher named Annie.

We were using the yoga room at my studio for the meeting. Annie told me she had two main problems with her teaching. One, she felt that her confidence was low, making her doubt herself. Two, her students often failed to cooperate, ignoring instructions, or doing something else. As Annie finished telling me about her challenges, she became emotional, and I empathized. However, as I listened to her, the problem was immediately obvious to me, but to be sure, I came up with a quick exercise. I set up three chairs across the room on three yoga mats. There was lots of space between each mat, one in the middle, the other two toward the sides of the room. I asked Annie to imagine she was teaching a class in this room, maybe 30 minutes into her sequence, and we chose a couple of postures (as she was a Hot Yoga teacher, we agreed on the Awkward Pose and Eagle). As Annie began teaching, she took a while to get into the slightly crazy and unfamiliar set up, pretending that three chairs on yoga mats were three students. But once she relaxed a little and made it more real, it started working well. The problem I sensed earlier still remained: Annie's voice was low. What I mean, when I say low is quiet and low in energy. Actually, waaaaaay too low for the size of the room we were in, and the intensity of the Awkward pose. I told Annie, "I like how courageous you are performing such an unfamiliar exercise and I like your instructions, they were precise! Now, we do have a problem but we can fix it. I felt that you spoke to yourself, rather than to your students. When you speak in a low volume, your voice does not leave your body and reach the students to 'shake up' and motivate them into the Awkward pose, before continuing strongly to get into the Eagle. Your low voice creates the impression that you're unsure what you want them to do and they don't have enough energy. You need to SPEAK LOUDER and STRONGER, so that your voice can reach the students, and even more importantly: fill the room. Let's do it again!"

After 15-20 minutes of trying to fill the room with her voice and failing, Annie got it right. As soon as she reached the correct volume, I stopped her, "That's it; you've got it!" Annie became emotional again. She said that she felt good speaking loudly—strong and sure of herself. At first, she thought she was too loud, but figured that if I didn't stop her or cover my ears, she would keep going. Haha.

So true! When you're learning to speak loudly but not used to it, you may feel as if it's too loud. If that's you, then you are too quiet.

Your voice must fill the room—it will make you a "better" teacher, and your students will subconsciously believe you to be a good teacher. The bigger the space, the more you will need to project your voice so that it fills the room. If you're in a huge room, like a conference hall, or teaching outside in a park, you will need a microphone and speaker system to help you. Nevertheless, the general rule for volume in group classes at an indoor location is this: the voice must fill the room.

Imagine a person speaking with the volume of his or her voice controlled by a remote control device in your hand. There is a volume setting on the remote that goes from 0 to 10. At volume 0, the person is silent. You turn up the volume to 1— they're speaking in a whisper. Volume 2—the whisper begins to be heard better; volume 3—they're speaking quietly. Volume 4 or 5, they're speaking like everyone else; normal voice, you can hear them as long as they're not far from you. Volume 6—you can hear them even if they turn around and are away from you. Volume 7—the voice begins to fill the room and at volume 8, the voice fills the room. Volume 9—they're speaking loudly, you worry that they may be angry with you. Volume 10 is extreme, good for shouting "Fire! Fire!"—or any other kind of emergency instruction.

Which volume setting do you think a yoga teacher should use when teaching a class? Volume 5 or 6? Nope. Volume 7 or 8 is the right level. Again, if you doubt what I say—you are too quiet.

How to Speak Louder

First of all, remember or re-read "The Stance and Breath" chapters. Keep in mind the correct breath, which we talked about, and an upright spine. You will know that the key to speaking louder is to have a lot of air reach your vocal cords before it exits your mouth. Let's do a quick exercise and you will get it. Hold a couple of fingers in front of your mouth, maybe a centimeter (half an inch) away. Count out loud from one to ten, get louder as you go along. At "1" you speak quietly, at "10" you finish very loudly. Ready? Don't forget the fingers. Let's count!

Did you feel more and more air hitting your fingers as you got louder? If you did, great—that's what we want. Perform this exercise a few more times until you get good at it. Once you're there, you will also feel more vibration in your vocal cords, which is good news.

A Reminder about Volume: On several occasions, I did some voice coaching for speakers who were hiding behind a small, constrained voice. When asked to speak louder, the usual response was "No, no! I'm already shouting!"

I've encouraged you more than once to stop saving your voice and let that energy out! Please stay with me on this: all your well-chosen instructions, pitch, vocal variation, and melody are not going to be of any use if people can't hear you in the first place.

Keep your volume up at 7 (and sometimes 8). This ensures that everyone in the room can hear you at all times. Even though you may be passing the corner of the room, facing away from the group, or at the back of the room, kneeling down to assist a student—keep your volume up to fill the room. There's nothing more unprofessional than speaking at a low volume so that students have to hold their breath to hear what's being said or guess what to do by following others nearer to the teacher.

Secondly, keeping your volume up is paramount for establishing yourself as a knowledgeable and competent teacher.

Thirdly, using volume 7 or 8 as your regular level will make you stand out compared to other quieter teachers (even those who have been teaching for years!)—you will be more popular, and when you acknowledge that fact, you will feel good.

Finally, volume 7 or 8 delivers energy and what we need is vibration—the voice resonates in the bodies of your students and vibrates in the walls of the building. It's bound to take a bit of courage on your part to discover "the new you," but when you do, it will blow you away.

What's next, once you've arrived at a good volume? Bring melody to the way you sound and tune the pitch of your voice.

MELODY AND PITCH

I t's time for you to discover what singers have known for a long time: melody can bring your words to life.

A while ago when I was designing my website, I got stuck on a technical glitch I couldn't solve. What I usually do in such cases is go to YouTube and look for a tutorial: a walk-through video, to learn how to solve the issue. Right from the beginning of the clip, the speaker starts in a low, monotone voice "Hello, my name is Jack and I'm here to walk you through the technical aspects of... blah blah blah." Thirty seconds into the clip, I'm already checking how long it is, knowing full well that I will not survive the dull delivery.

When someone speaks in a monotone way, we tune out. We stop listening, and science backs this up. We subconsciously tune people out because the monotone is too predictable. We can guess what the person is going to say next. If your students are conscious of this, here's what they are likely to tell you as the monotone-speaking trainer, "We realize that we are hearing the same note over and over again. So after perhaps half a minute, we already know which sounds you are about to make." You're in trouble when this happens. "If we think we know the sound you're going to make, we tune you out and stop listening. We simply imagine the words you're going to say before you say them. We don't bother to pay attention. After all, if we already know the ending of the story, why should we listen to the middle?"

In an effective yoga teacher's voice, we would look for a high level of melody (lots of intonation), so everyone will know that you have an exciting, interesting personality and can bring a lot of knowledge to the table. Continuous melody shows lots of color, enthusiasm toward work, and a zest for life. There's absolutely no room here for the teacher or instructor to sound as dull as dishwater.

Please work on the assumption that most people have a surprisingly short attention span. If they think they already know what you're going to say, the conversation is pretty much over. The goal is to use melody in your voice to create variation and keep them guessing. If your voice moves up and down like the melody of a good song, it will become like their favorite tune.

To help you get started with melody, the simplest plan is this:

- Learn to vary your intonation.
- During your melody practice, use your hands a bit more than usual.
- Keep your volume up.

I have a couple of exercises to make sure you are not one of those monotone yoga teachers.

The first exercise is a bit crazy. You'll have to trust me a little, but it will immediately improve your tonality and get you to achieve melody++ (I pronounce this "melody plus plus", meaning lots of melody.) Please, sing the Happy Birthday song out loud. I can imagine you saying to yourself "no way." Go on, please. "Happy birthday to you... Happy birthday to you... Happy birthday, dear Julie—happy birthday to youuu..."

Melody++, yes? Good. Now, sing your yoga posture or other exercise instructions to the same tune. Try it with me. Sing: "Feet together, strong legs... Bring your arms up overhead... Take a big step to the ri–ight—and open your armzz..."

Got it? That's melody! That's what we want. That's how to tune into the level of variation you're putting into your voice.

For the second exercise, choose a passage from a book or magazine and record yourself reading out loud. Play the recording back, and listen specifically for how high and low you go. Does your voice go up and down and everywhere in between, or does it sound like Jack the YouTube instructor? I encourage you to move your voice around as you speak. Introduce lots of variety and give it plenty of melody. As you experiment in this way, you'll no doubt come up with a lot of "goofy" sounds and little voices you may never use. But you'll also stumble upon certain qualities you like and want to incorporate. You'll get the best results if you spend time to consciously exaggerate the highs and lows, and move into areas you're not used to exploring.

The next time you are teaching, listen to yourself. If you catch yourself in the monotone or any kind of usual-slightly-boring pattern, bring melody++ into it and watch your students' eyes light up. That is the sign of interest; that is attention—exactly what we want.

The trick is to keep surprising. That's the main use of melody. What surprises your listeners is that you're able to make them feel a certain way: energized, thoughtful, relaxed, restored, or any number of other emotional states beneficial to your content. Remember, one of the reasons why you are reading this book is to make changes in your career and perhaps your life, yes? If you can have more control over the way others feel when within reach of your voice, you're much closer to your goal. I would like you to get rid of the boring, monotone voice you used to have once and for all. Swap it for the voice that brings excitement, variety, mystery, fun, and energy. Having more melody is a great way to make that happen.

Watch out for Finishing on a Low Tone

Have you ever tried to send a child to sleep with a story? Imagine telling the story line by line and at the end of each one, you lower the tone of your voice then start the next line at the deep tone you ended on. So your voice drops down and down, like walking down the stairs one step at a time.

When you finish each line on a low tone, your voice has an impact on the listener, telling their body to relax, and their breath and heart rate to slow down. It is not the story that sends the child to sleep, but the sound (tonality) of your voice—it does the job at a deeper level. And you might have seen a magician or hypnotist, who puts the audience to sleep in seconds with their down-down tonality.

Importantly, I must tell you of one more downward tonality

that many instructors have. This one has added loudness, with the body pacing up and down in the yoga room. The pacing (walking back and forth, often shuffling the feet a bit) creates overconfidence and brings more air into the lungs. The instructor's brain function is faster as it receives more oxygen. But the extra volume in the lungs gives a loud, forceful, downward inflection, which may sound too commanding, especially when mixed with exercises filled with adrenaline ("high energy"). Certain students will be attracted to the strong leadership indicated by the downward-tone, loud-volume voice since they feel reassured that whatever danger may be hiding around the corner, the instructor is capable of handling it. Therefore, they feel safe. Unfortunately, for the majority of practitioners, such a leadership voice is too aggressive and looney. It seems to them that the instructor is responding strongly to the imagined threat, but the group simply doesn't see it. In consequence, they don't trust the instructor and will leave as soon as it is possible, or polite, to do so.

Watch out for a High Pitch

Although we want lots of melody, we don't want to go high-pitched (thin) like Minnie Riperton. Look her up on YouTube and you will know what I mean.

The thinner the sound of my voice, the more likely the people around me will find it irritating and the less likely they are to take me seriously. Of course, there's a wide variety in what sounds we, as individuals, find appealing, but in general terms, a high-pitched nasal voice is much less pleasant to listen to than a lower pitch, resonant one, rich in undertones. Stay on the lower side of the pitch, but not too low—that will keep you out of trouble.

Mix Volume and Melody

The key now is to mix these two. When you teach a class, vary the volume and melody of your voice in such a way so as not to appear mad and angry, but interesting. You must discover your own way of mixing, and find your own style where you can sound strong and confident when necessary, or happy, enthusiastic, and nourishing. That way, you are much more likely to get out of the monotone and keep the close attention of your class.

PACE

"You can tell how nervous I am by how fast I am talking," said Catherine Deneuve, a superstar actress of the 70s.

Have you ever taken a Bikram Hot Yoga class? Every time I've gone into one, I've been hit by the vocal machine gun delivery of the instructor. It's a bit like being run over by a train. The delivery is absolutely relentless, and after a while it's impossible to follow. You're thinking about leaving, and perhaps against your better judgment, you let the instructor keep going, though you may have to step outside for a moment at the end to stop your head from spinning. You may also come across the fast-paced horse racing commentaries and television commercials. When you hear this kind of ultra-fast talking, what are you thinking? You most likely make an assumption that the speaker is trying to project a sense of urgency and importance. Subconsciously, you may also feel that they are nervous or hiding something.

When leading a class, what does your pace tell others about you? And how does the pace affect what they hear? Keep in mind that we all "run" at a different speed. If I am high-strung and restless, my metabolism may be, by my nature, set on high. I walk briskly, eat quickly, and speak fast. And vice versa, someone could have a calm deposition, patient, centered, and grounded, never appearing to be in a hurry. Their heart rate is usually slower, with extended breathing.

Let's see how we can find out about your natural speed. Do you talk slower than the people around you? Faster? Spend some time being curious and aware of how your pace compares with that of others around you. I'm not saying there's a "good" or "bad" pace—just trying to get a feel for it.

We can play with pacing the speed of your voice as you talk. Let's start by you picking up a magazine or book and reading from it into your recording app. First, read two or three sentences at your normal speed. Then, change the pace: slow down for another sentence or two. Then, speed up again. Which pace sounds best in your opinion? Which one makes you sound exciting to listen to, powerfully energizing, or compassionate and calming? Please realize that, verbally, various parts of your teaching will be more (and less!) effective at different paces of speech. There's no golden rule here. Generally speaking, I find that more energizing instructions need to be given faster than normal. Slowing down is more relaxing to listen to, of course, but again, the key here is to learn to speak slower, normal, and faster according to your needs and the visible response of the people in front of you. As you're teaching, when you speak slowly you take the risk that your voice will make you sound lazy, disinterested, or sluggish. It would be a different matter, however, if you were leading a guided meditation, for example.

The important thing is to be comfortable, and definitely not to speak too fast. It is good to have variety in pace: use it like the gas pedal in your car. You would never drive at 50 kilometers per hour for a whole trip. As you teach, it is good to speed up at the more energizing or encouraging moments, but be able to slow down and let the students rest. As my teacher Jimmy Barkan always pointed out, it is also good to keep things "conversational." When we're involved in a conversation, we can vary our talking pace naturally. We can do the same when leading a class, which sounds good indeed.

Think of vocal pace as both the speed of speech and the number of instructions/ideas per minute. If you are a naturally high-energy, fast speaker you will feel uncomfortable slowing down. In this case, I would suggest you make lots of pauses (to be discussed later). Your students will have a chance to listen and coordinate your verbal cues, before you slam them with the next burst of a hundred instructions per minute.

The best way to find the right pace is through trial and error. There's no magic pill for fixing the pace of your speech, just speak, observe, and adjust. Use the recording app on your phone for practice. Bear in mind that various teaching situations require a different pace.

Once you're teaching "live", the key is to create an even pace, allowing the class to follow your material without getting bored and distracted by anything else. You may go a little faster than usual. If the practice is supposed to be energizing, by keeping your vocal pace up you are challenging the class to keep up with you. On the other hand, when you want to achieve relaxation or cool down, you may slow your vocal pace down. Slow is not inherently bad. Be sure that it is complimenting what you want to achieve—your class will let you know. Observe them carefully and see how they respond to the changes in pace.

ARTICULATION

In this book, I focus on teaching classes in English, but if you teach in another language, it's quite easy to do a little extra research on your own. Search the Internet for the equivalent of "diction" or "articulation" in your own language and find a few good resources.

The common meaning of diction (articulation) according to Wiki is, "the distinctiveness of speech, the art of speaking so that each word is clearly heard and understood to its fullest complexity and extremity, and concerns pronunciation and tone, rather than word choice and style. This secondary sense is more precisely and commonly expressed with the term enunciation, or with its synonym articulation."

When we consider teaching in English, I often find that a British speaker has the most difficulty with diction. This is largely due to how the sounds of the English language are produced in the mouth, especially by the main active articulators; the tongue and lower lip. In general, spoken English does not require the use of the tongue or lips as much as other languages. Have you seen upper class English speakers on YouTube? Take my long-time favorite, John Cleese. His mouth hardly opens and moves at all when he speaks. Go ahead, discover for yourself. Go to YouTube and search for Monty Python, John Cleese.

Suffice to say, whatever your particular culture, language, or upbringing—most common diction issues are solved by speaking loudly (volume 7!). It is difficult to mumble, when speaking at volume 7—try it for yourself!

There is a super easy and cool exercise for practicing your diction or articulation. I call it the nightclub exercise. Have you ever been to a nightclub? What? Are you laughing at me? You think it's a silly question—of course you've been to a night club. Let me digress for a moment before I come back to the articulation part. Some years ago, I was teaching in Indonesia. I was hired to train six young Pilates instructors to teach Hot Yoga classes. During the first week, we got onto the subject of articulation. My small group was sitting in front of me in a circle and I asked them a "rhetorical" question, "Have you ever been to a nightclub?" expecting, of course, that they had. But I can see them shaking their heads. No, they had never been to a nightclub! They were all in their early twenties, and in Indonesia, you just don't do any nightclubbing at that age. Haha. After this, I learned not to take anything for granted. So in case that you haven't been to a nightclub either let me tell you that the place is packed with people. The music speakers are pumping so loud that nobody can hear anything else. When you're there with a friend and you ask them if they want another drink, if you speak normally, they will not hear you. So the way to do it is to get them to look at you and "read your lips." You will articulate, actually, you will OVER articulate the words in such a way that your friend can guess what you're saying.

The above method of over-articulation is a great exercise to improve your diction. In an over–articulated tone: Practice speaking as if you are in a nightclub, talking to a friend who cannot hear what you are saying, so has to read your lips. Have fun with this.

TAKE OUT THE FILLERS

In the mistaken belief that silence is bad during teaching, we worry unnecessarily that we may lose our students' attention. In reality, silence allows the group to process and coordinate what they have just heard. Here are some hints on how to eliminate "ummms" and "errs," "I mean, like...," "so...," "you know..."

Firstly, embrace the silence. Take advantage of the commas and periods in your instructions and make no sound when they occur, rather than subscribing to the all–to–common habit of filling them with ummms and errrs, or other connecting sounds. At a comma, let your voice go up in tone slightly, pause, then return to the rest of the sentence. The students will expect you to return to the sentence because your voice went up. That way, you will gain the necessary courage to leave even bigger pauses whenever you want.

Secondly, learn to connect all the words together as you speak. Many instructors don't know how to do that, and create a poor impression. All words need to be connected together on a single, underlying beam of air. Use melody to connect all the words together in a way that is pleasing for the listener. Basically:

speakallthewordsconnectingthemtogetheruntilyougettoa-comma—STOP—

connectthenewgroupofwordsspeakingmoreuntilyouge-tothenextcomma—STOP

You will notice the improvement immediately.

PAUSES

We tend to worry that pausing will create a bad impression. Perhaps the reason we are afraid to pause is because we think it shows hesitation, and we haven't figured out what to say. We may be concerned about appearing a slow talker, making us look and sound unprepared and inarticulate. This may well be the case if I am naturally a super-slow talker: when I speak super slowly, I'm at risk of pausing too often, as if I want to make it easy for my students to understand. The individual ideas or instructions will be too disconnected—making it easy to lose track. I'm also more likely to start filling the pauses with errrs and ummms (called "fillers," as mentioned earlier). When I am listening to a super-slow speaking instructor, and even worse, one who makes frequent pauses, I find myself questioning their competence. The pauses seem to be signs of hesitation, my subconscious suggesting a lack of authority.

As long as you are not a super-slow speaker, able to vary

and adjust your pace as required, I believe pauses are necessary and important. When I teach my yoga class, I like to tell my students that yoga is not in the poses, it's in the pauses. The pauses you make give you time to breathe and your students the chance to breathe mentally and coordinate the actions of the yoga asanas. The pauses allow everyone to observe, to listen, to digest, to say, "Hmmmm... that's interesting," before getting ready for more action.

Think of using pauses like punctuation: a short pause for a comma, longer pause for a full stop (period), and an even longer pause in between paragraphs.

If the pauses are not there, the teacher's energy is exhausted and he or she is unable to see what's in front of them; meanwhile, the students are becoming frustrated, even to the point of anger, that they don't have time to carry out the instructions.

Lack of pauses may be one of the most common reasons why students leave the room in the middle of a class.

In my professional opinion, few teachers pause for long enough. It seems that those who do apply pauses properly took years to reach that point. Perhaps this is because when we are nervous or excited our sense of timing is erratic. What in reality is only a second often feels like eight when teaching a room full of students. So pauses are rarely long enough.

We need to give clear spaces between chunks of instructions —very clear, obvious spaces; for example, "Downward facing dog. Set your hands shoulder distance apart and spread your fingers wide. Feet pointing directly forward, set them about hip distance apart. As you press away from the floor through the arms, lengthen your spine. Breathe evenly through your nose and stay there for three more breaths—PAUSE. Now step forward on the right foot between your hands, warrior number one..." Avoid being subtle. When you're learning to pause during a class, the pauses must be longer than feels comfortable to you.

I once met a woman in my Hot Yoga teacher training course who, like many others during the first week, was absolutely terrified of standing up in front of others during the mock classes. Then, as often happens, in the second or third week she found her voice and by week four, she could not stop talking. Even when teaching the softer, restorative postures, she would continue to deliver instructions like a machine gun! I wanted her to pause, she wanted to pause too, but could not. So I came up with an idea—she had to hold a water bottle when giving instructions. The exercise was to say two or three pieces of instruction—pause to take a sip of water—say three more instructions— sip the water—and so forth. You see, the trick works, because it is difficult to successfully drink and speak at the same time, and when you try it in front of others, you don't want to embarrass yourself by starting to choke up and cough! Pause to take a sip of water. Try this yourself when you need to. It works wonders.

Once, I traveled with a friend of mine and his young kid, a boy. Together, we watched the same in-flight movie. When the movie was finished, the boy said he liked it, because "the people in the movie didn't talk much, so he understood more."

The pauses must not be subtle. Make them clear and obvious. That's what the yoga guru B.K.S. Iyengar may have meant when he said, "When you stop speaking, the students start listening." You see, few of us listen a hundred percent of the time to anyone; our minds wander. It's the way it is, we know that. So we're going to use the pauses to bring the students' attention back and for that reason, they will love your pauses and your class. Now, their minds will be thinking "Yippee, I'm back in the zone. I know where I am. Thank you."

One more important note about a common problem: are you running out of breath before the end of the sentence, or even earlier? Whenever there's a comma, there's an inhale to go with it. Put more commas into your sentences if necessary. The problem is incorrect breathing—most likely you're not using diaphragm-based breath and not taking in enough air. Please note that when you speak louder, you use less air, not more. Speak louder so that you don't run out of breath.

Debussy, one of the great composers, said that music is the space between the notes. Invite your students to put in a quiet pause between each breath, experience the space between the breaths—the space between the thoughts—it's where yoga happens.

USING SILENCE

"Immerse yourself in silence," said the Bulgarian mystic O.M. Aivanhov, "Abandon yourself to the embrace of silence as a child abandons itself to the embrace of its mother's arms, and harmony will grow within you and reach into every smallest cell of your body."

I want to tell you something personal. It took me years to realize that a yoga class is perhaps not about teaching asana, even though that's what I do—it's about creating the possibility that participants can experience something special. By selflessly focusing on the students in the present moment, the teacher is allowing enough space for them to experience the power, magic, and benefits of yoga at their own pace and according to their own needs.

I believe that most students do not come to the class for yoga. They are looking for help. They want to improve their health, self-esteem, take a break from being under pressure, or perhaps they're looking for a way out of an emotional or spiritual crisis. A good yoga teacher is blessed with the opportunity to create an experience of well-being and inspiration for the students.

In terms of teaching a yoga class, what is the difference between a pause and silence? Silence is a long pause.

In my class, silence creates a space for stillness. When there's stillness in silence and silence in stillness, the space is open for your students to directly experience harmony. I stress the importance of this: make sure that in each and every class you teach, there are at least five minutes of stillness at the end. The real power of absolute stillness is often underestimated. In stillness, everything comes together for your students. As the central nervous system slows down, the undisturbed body is able to embrace the benefits of the previous exercises. Stillness is important to enable healing to take place. It is awesome for stress-release. I bring all this into the final relaxation at the end of the practice.

To begin the final Savasana, you can let your students lay down on the yoga mat and relax for a minute. Then try this, it works wonders: give some pointers using only one sentence at a time. Lower the pitch of your voice and speak slowly, with plenty of silent moments in between lines. Sit cross-legged among your students, keeping a straight spine. Be present, empathize, enjoy. The magic of teaching yoga is active when your students get a taste of samadhi in the final relaxation and you are there to share in their achievement, to savor it.

PART IV

VOICE SKILLS

MY EXPERIENCE WITH TEACHERS

I'm bringing you some brief case histories relating to the voice, each of which I have experienced in my coaching work with yoga.

One female instructor from Singapore who works with me now over Skype does so because, since she started teaching a year ago, she never felt that she would have enough breath to support her voice and class demonstrations. She says, "There is never any relief; every breath is a struggle for me. It is discouraging to know that my students can hear me fighting with my breath in every class I teach." After chatting for a while on the Internet video, it became clear to me that she has never done any basic breath-work for speaking—none at all. It was not a part of her teacher training, and she had no previous experience with public speaking or singing. We had to start at the beginning with stance and breath. As her posture and breathing improved, she began to discover her natural voice, and this felt satisfying, to say the least. The problem was that no foundation had been laid out in the training program on which to build her voice. Only by admitting to herself that things weren't working and having the courage to seek help, can she now improve.

I helped out a young but experienced Pilates instructor attending my Hot Yoga teacher training class in Indonesia. Whenever it was necessary to speak louder (and you must remember that I coach teachers to speak at volume 7), she would go higher in both volume and pitch. She would be speaking loudly, in a squeaky, thin voice—it was incredibly annoying. Everyone else in the room would immediately frown and back away from her, or even cover their ears. I think the reason for that unbearable pitch was nervousness. It was a challenge for her to speak loudly (as a Muslim female, loudness may not have been part of her culture). Being required to speak in front of others in her Pilates class was fine, as she would usually teach one or two students in a small room. Preparing to teach a well-attended Hot Yoga class in a large space requires the volume to be kept up. The high pitch was finally resolved when she learned to speak in such a way that her voice would resonate deeply in her chest (lower pitch), instead of the nose and forehead (high pitch).

Then there was the yoga teacher in Bangkok, who would frequently lose her voice. Actually, she was one of many overworked instructors in the company she worked for. Being forced to teach too many classes, there was never enough time to rest her voice. But most interesting to me was that always the same teachers tended to lose their voice. Others were fine, even though they also taught for long hours. Although I had no way of finding out for sure about the others, this particular person was a "mouth breather." You could hear it as soon as she began to increase the volume and pace. When speaking normally during a conversation, she was fine. Speaking in class demanded more volume and speed—she would take the inhales through her mouth. Her voice box began to dry up, eventually, her voice became scratchy—she would need to start clearing her throat more often, then began coughing. Eventually, her voice would be gone for three or four days, which would force her to take time off, without pay. Luckily, I was able to spot the inhales through the mouth. Once the problem was identified, she needed to practice reading loudly from a book to an imaginary audience, focusing on inhales through the nose. I'm sure you know that the nasal passages moisten the air before it reaches the voice strings, which is crucial for healthy speech, especially when talking a lot at high "energy."

For any yoga teacher, losing their voice is bad news. In the next chapter, let's find out how to take care of your voice better.

HOW TO DEMONSTRATE AND SPEAK

Having to occasionally perform the postures as we are speaking is one area of our work we cannot avoid. For many fast practicing yoga teachers (fast vinyasa-style teachers, for example), the job requires a combination of movement and voice work. Unfortunately, physical performance and a good voice don't work well together. I have a tip for you to ease the problem: rehearse beforehand. To become proficient at exercising and relaying instructions at the same time you need to rehearse prior to going "live." Look for parts of the sequence where you may be losing your voice due to lack of breath, the failure to keep a good stance, or any other compromising position where your voice is not projecting well.

When you speaking while in a pose, the danger area is in those postures where the breath is shallow; twists for instance (or postures similar to the Cobra). For fast practices, most voice projection problems occur as the teacher is out of breath due to the intensity of the exercise. Even though slightly out-of-breath-

and-speaking may be good for a short time in providing energy, beware of long periods where you're likely to lose your voice if speaking without having adequate breath beyond the exhale, and/or breathing in through the mouth.

If you plan carefully, your voice will not be damaged and with real-time experience, movement and speech will seamlessly integrate. Without preparation, you may not last more than a week of intense teaching. With forward preparation, your body, actions, breath, and voice can all work in unison, keeping your vocal cords in good condition and safe from strain.

VOICE CARE

Drink plenty of water. I suggest you drink at least eight large glasses a day, and even more, if you're a big fella or gal. Drink even more water if you live in a dry climate, or live and teach in air-conditioned spaces. Water is essential for a good voice because hydration brings moisture to the vital voice organs. The cords in the voice box vibrate as you're speaking (I read somewhere that the voice strings vibrate even when we're asleep, dreaming about speaking. Crazy!). Check to see the color of your urine. If it's pale, you're well hydrated. The darker your urine, the more problems will occur with your voice. Avoid drinking cold water. It cools down your voice—it works best warm. Speaking for a living naturally, means the voice is used a lot. Talking may irritate the voice strings quite a bit, but when we drink plenty of water, some useful phlegm will be secreted to coat them. Drinking lots of water on a daily basis is the best voice care advice I can give you.

Stop smoking. Not only is it bad for your health, but for your voice too. If you're not able to quit, at least cut down. If you quit, you may have a few weeks of struggling with extra mucus, then your voice will be clear and sound good.

If you smoke marihuana, since it burns at a high temperature, it is damaging to your voice strings. You will be better off smoking it through a hookah; a type of water pipe.

If you are emotionally going through a hard time, the pain will show up in your voice. It may be necessary to take a break from teaching and return to work when you feel better.

Many people have a habit of regularly clearing their throats. Not a good thing. You need to work with a relaxed throat, get good at swallowing saliva easy. Alcohol, coffee, cola-type drinks, eating dairy and red meat late in the evening—all are bad news —they will make you want to clear your throat.

I recommend avoiding aspirin for a cold or sore throat; choose an aspirin-free painkiller instead. Be careful with mucus-reducing medication and lozenges (eucalyptus, menthol, etc.). Although these will dry the excess mucus, they are likely to create voice problems if taken within a few hours of teaching a class.

Here are a few more tips for voice care:

- Avoid speaking more than twelve hours in one day.
- Do not smoke and avoid breathing in secondhand smoke.
- Avoid caffeine and other diuretics (coffee, tea, cola, etc.).
- Avoid eating and drinking products containing refined sugar.
- Avoid chewing gum.

- Avoid lemon and other citrus (acid type) fruits.
- Cut down on alcoholic drinks.
- Avoid lozenges and throat sprays.
- Avoid consuming hot or cold drinks before taking a class.
- Get at least seven to eight hours of sleep daily.

If you find yourself without a choice, and working with a strained voice, try to get a hands-free microphone.

If that's not possible, and you're still going ahead with the idea of teaching with a weakened voice, have an assistant or a colleague tell your class beforehand that you have a problem. That way, if you're making strange vocal sounds, your students will be more forgiving. In my own experience, they may even enjoy your class more. Something about knowing that their teacher is human, perhaps even vulnerable, may help them appreciate you. Speak much less than you usually would and at a lower pitch. Pace yourself.

OVERCOMING NERVOUSNESS AND ANXIETY

When you get nervous or anxious, it may be normal for the pace of your voice to go into super-fast mode and/or lose its charm. Perhaps your voice sounds great one-on-one, or in a familiar situation with people you know well. But when you stand in front of a group of students, adrenaline kicks in and your heart rate goes up, and if you can't find a way to calm yourself, it's guaranteed your words will rush out way too fast, like bullets from a machine gun. Even worse, the sound of your voice will suffer. You could end up losing all of the colorful melody you have learned. Instead, you may fall back into the hopeless monotone voice. When teaching, if we rush through the instructions to our students without giving ourselves time to breathe, there is little chance our voices will produce the best possible sound. So what should we do?

Please understand that speaking in public is one of our most critical fears. "We are more afraid of public speaking than we are of dying," my hero Jerry Seinfeld said, "Which means that if there's a funeral, I'd rather be the guy in the coffin than the man speaking the eulogy." On the upside, overcoming the fear is a tremendously satisfying AND life-changing experience.

"Stage fright" is one of the most misunderstood gifts your body can present you with. That fear connects to your fight-or-flight reflex (i.e. the sympathetic nervous system). You can use the magnificent amount of energy which comes with that response to improve your performance! Here's what to do: assign a new name to your stage fright—call it something more positive. Then, connect the fresh surge of energy to your work in that moment, but do not allow your breathing pattern to change, or if it does, then make sure it's not more than a little. Extend each breath: breathe deeper and slower—you will feel like a rock star.

I have one more awesome technique to support you in times of stage fright. Keeping your hands level with your waistline is one of the most effective ways to effortlessly resist the stress of public speaking. When your hands are placed low; level with your waist but not down, how you look and sound will be sending messages to your students that you are an expert, calm and competently in charge. What's more, they will feel that you are authentic and trustworthy. Try it!

PART V

WORKING SPACE

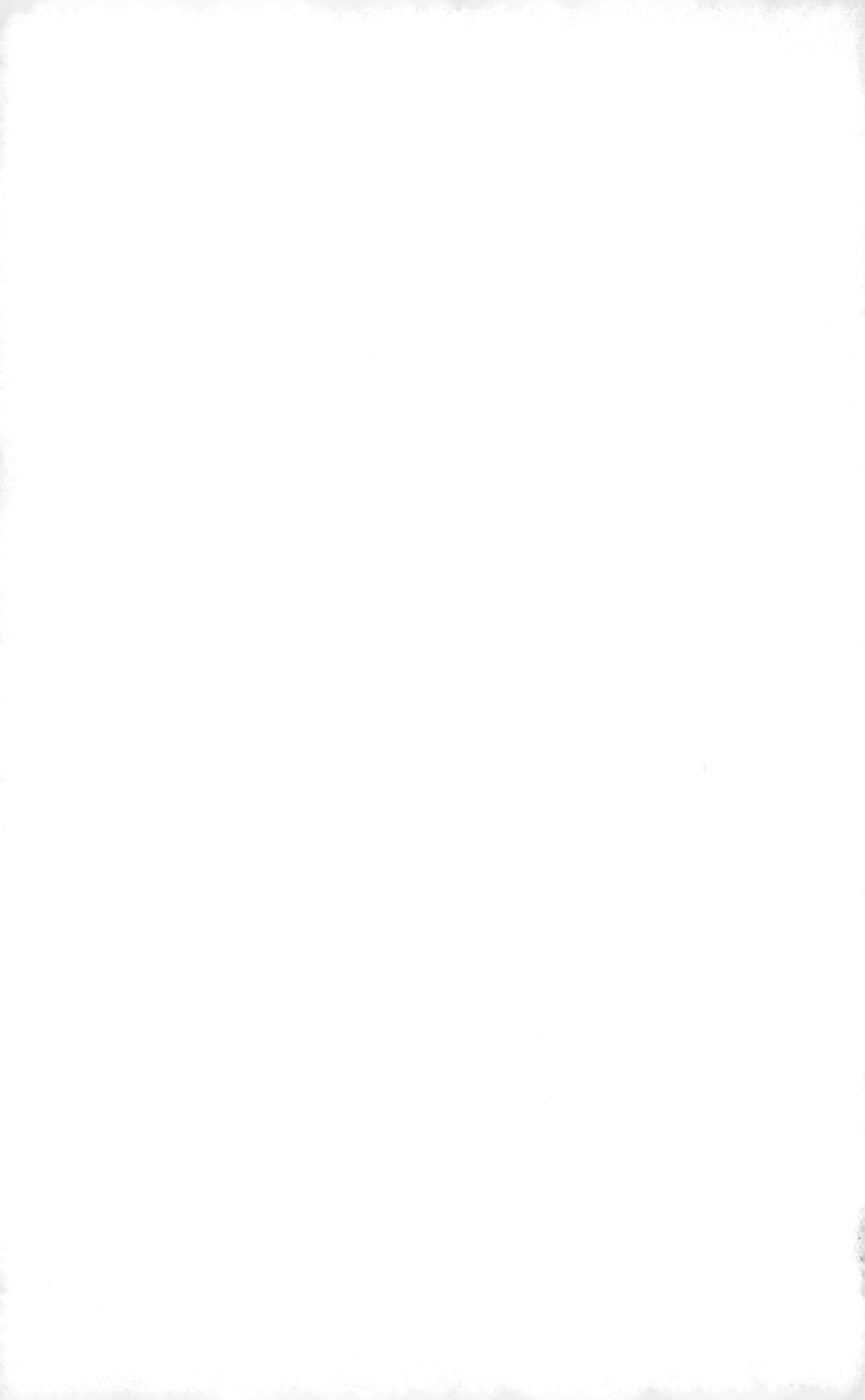

TEACHING SPACE

Prince, the famous rock star, passed away recently. He wrote a song called "Vicki Waiting," and part of the lyrics went something like this:

I told the joke about the woman
Who asked her lover "Why is your organ so small?"
He replied, "I didn't know I was playin' in a cathedral."

One of the biggest challenges for a yoga teacher has to do with working in various locations, each with a different space. Not only does the space change its energy dynamics depending on the number of persons in the room, but each space will place different demands on your voice. This depends on the space's size and type of acoustics.

I will try to define some important pointers for you regarding teaching classes or sessions in different spaces. Teachers who wouldn't usually bother with working space considerations may find that the acoustics will overwhelm their voices and defeat their performance.

"DEAD OR ALIVE?"

When you're teaching at a new location, you need to test the space. Just like an actor or singer, you want to find out if it's acoustically dead or alive. If you say loudly "HA!", and the voice comes back to you like a tiny echo, that space is alive. Check how quiet you can be before you're too quiet. Check how loud you can speak before you're too loud. Dead spaces give you no feedback—your voice will need more projection. A live space needs more articulation, more mini-pauses between words, and a bit less volume.

LARGE SPACES

The larger the space you are teaching your class in, the more breath you will need—which is why I recommend that before teaching live in an unfamiliar space, you arrive early and "breathe" the space so you can get a better idea of the challenges you face.

You must articulate more. You will need to keep your volume up, especially at the end of each line (sentence). All syllables will need to be spoken clearly, which may feel a bit strange to you, but it will be appreciated by your people. If you have a strong accent, in large spaces it may need to be adjusted to provide less twang and more definition.

It will be more difficult to be heard if you move around a lot. In a big room, you may find it necessary to stay in one place when speaking, move, and then speak in one place again. Your body and voice will need to come together even more than in a small or regular space.

People may be looking at your face more often than in small spaces. If you turn away from them, they may easily be lost.

You will need to project more energy; this will obviously require lots of volume, but also melody—otherwise, you risk sounding angry. You may need to speak slower and less frequently than usual.

Louder? Yes! But don't shout or push your voice too much. If you speak too loudly, people will become oblivious to what you're saying. They can hear you but will stop listening to the content. You're also certain to lose your voice.

It's easy to be intimidated by a large space if you're not used to working in one. Don't be. Get there early. Breathe the space deeply. Walk around, place your hand on the wall—own it.

It's good to teach in large working spaces. You know that your voice needs to meet the challenge, and this will inspire you. It's easy to get lazy teaching in small spaces. But you need to own the big space with your voice. If your students cannot hear you, they will be upset and unforgiving.

SMALL SPACES

The problem with small working spaces is that you may get vocally lazy: your students are close to you, so your voice skills don't have to be in the game.

Another problem is energy: in a small space, it will be difficult for you to project your voice in an energized way. You will feel inhibited and claustrophobic. Actually, I think that for high-energy yoga classes, small working spaces should be avoided.

When you're working in a small space, get there early to test it. Check how high your voice can go before it's too loud.

When you're working in a small room, get your voice to fill the room (as discussed earlier in the "Volume" chapter). Small spaces have an intimate feel to them. If your voice is good and resonates in the walls, your people (and you!) will enjoy being there.

OUTDOOR SPACES

You will need lots of breath.

You will need to finish your words and lines.

But there are even more challenges here, and they're external. Open spaces are subject to the wind, causing trees to rustle. The wind will also dissipate your voice.

If you're turning your face or moving around a lot as you speak, your voice will not adequately reach your students. You will need to be still more when projecting your voice outdoors.

Beware of traffic noises, bird noises, and other noises in the distance.

Your voice may not have any reinforcement, unless your outdoor venue is in the corner between two walls or buildings, or you can use a wireless microphone and speakers.

NOISY SPACES

As a visiting teacher, I was recently teaching a yoga class in an unfamiliar place; a shala on the top floor of a two-story spa building with a high, pyramid-shaped roof. I would usually have gone early and "scouted" the location prior to teaching, but this time it wasn't possible—I was a last minute replacement for someone who had lost his voice.

It was a group yoga class, everything was going well. Then the rain came. In Thailand, where I live, when it rains—it pours. As the rain hit the roof, it sounded as if all hell had broken loose. The noise was overpowering but I decided to continue with the class. At that point, the only way to teach was to demonstrate—speaking wasn't working. I had to use a sort of improvised sign language to get the job done. It was bad. It was fun.

We may often encounter noise during our work, although perhaps not as extreme as in the situation above. When you find yourself teaching somewhere noisy, you will appreciate your voice craft. Good stance and good breath can give you extra support for speaking louder when necessary. Good articulation can help you to be understood as you speak louder. When you speak loudly in order to overcome a noisy environment, please remember to use lots of melody—otherwise, your students will be overpowered by the high volume, its energy may be too strong. Melody should soften that.

If you end up teaching in a place where the noise comes and goes in waves, you may need to time your instructions to speak in the quieter moments.

PART VI

BONUS MATERIALS

1

USING A MICROPHONE

Yoga studios and yoga rooms are becoming larger, classes are getting bigger, with outdoor classes gaining in popularity. Consequently, the use of a speaker system to amplify the teacher's voice has become more of a necessity than ever.

There are a few potential problems you should be aware of:

The microphone can expose vocal flaws in the most ruthless way. Every inhale you take will be amplified (and God help you if you're inhaling through your mouth). Every non-word sound—gasp, gulp, sigh, and vocal tic will be heard too. This means that if you're going to use the mic, your vocal technique must be even better. Hopefully, with this course under your belt, you've got what it takes.

You may be uncomfortable having the mic, the battery pack and wires attached to your face and body. Please also remember that the mic stays on unless you switch it off. If you need to go to the bathroom or have a private conversation (with yourself?)

and forget to switch off your mic, you may get into an embar-rassing situation.

Hearing your own voice amplified can be a shock. We know how we sound unplugged, but when our voice travels through electronic equipment and comes back at us, it can sound differ-ent. It changes with every step down the highway of cables, amps, and speakers (Half-jokingly, I tell the trainee teachers in my courses that the only "truth" occurs in the space between their mouth and the microphone.).

In my experience, teaching yoga classes with a microphone works best when the sound or vocal technique doesn't change merely for the sake of the electronics. My advice is not to speak in a softer or quieter way when you hear your voice amplified. Many people tend to do so as soon as they put on their headset microphone to test the sound. They may incorrectly assume that because the mic is doing all the work, the voice doesn't need to. Feel free to disagree. But as you know by now, a soft voice can't provide the energy necessary for the students to get through the class, so whether with a microphone or without, you need to keep your own volume up, okay? Does this mean you should use volume 7 directly into the microphone? No. You can adjust the volume coming through the sound system by changing how close the microphone is to your lips or using the volume control on the amplifier.

If your technique is now good and you have lots of breath to support your voice, you may not need a microphone at all. When I teach a regular class of 30 to 50 persons in a mid-sized setting, I'm okay without one. Many yoga rooms have good acoustics and the unamplified sound bounces off the walls and ceiling, creating a good experience. Of course, in a large hall or outdoors on a windy day, it's another story—a microphone and speakers will be needed.

The bottom line? Don't change your voice for the microphone. Allow yourself to use the volume you worked hard to develop. If necessary, use the microphone as an aid—not a reason for reverting to a soft, "lazy" voice.

2

THE INNER VOICE

Inner voices can be either your enemy or best supporters. There is a way of transforming negative inner chatter into a positive, uplifting force. We have all experienced an inner voice in our head, saying things like "You're not good enough for this," "Everyone will think you're a fake," "Do yourself a favor and quit right now." To be effective and successful as teachers, we need to learn to ignore and eventually eliminate that voice.

We also hear external voices. Our fellow teachers, yoga studio managers, students, opinions from social media—they all have something to say on the subject of our teaching.

3

INWARD CONFIDENCE

In order to address all the internal and external voices and opinions, I offer you the concept of "internal confidence, outward attention." It will be easier for you to feel internally confident and outwardly focused when you learn to forget about yourself. Remember that you are only the messenger. You are offering a service: information. It is not about you. In this way, when your tricky inner voice starts to speak and sabotages your confidence, you will realize that it's full of nonsense. Instead, suggest to yourself internally:

1. Your students are waiting to hear what you have to say.

2. They need to hear you.

3. Once they have heard you, their lives are going to change for the better.

When you bring this inner voice with you when it's time to lead a class, before you get started, mentally go through the three points; I guarantee you will find them helpful, and the way toward "inward confidence."

Confidence is not the goal here—being able to boost your inner confidence will consequently enable you to be more dynamic and communicate with ease, and that's what we want. It's also good to do some preparations. Here's a checklist I use for myself, and since it works so well, I've been sharing it with my teacher trainees. Now, I share it with you. When you are getting ready to teach a class, mentally go through this list (have it printed or saved in your phone):

1. My students love to hear me speak. That's because I've taken the time to work on my voice.

2. I feel and look good.

3. I will focus my mind on internal confidence and outward attention. I am here for my students to help them make good choices in their lives. This is not about me.

You may want to go through this checklist several times before you teach a class. Once you feel more confident, you can being to pay attention to what is happening around you.

4

OUTWARD ATTENTION

We're nearing the end of this book. During your work, as you lead your students through the sequence of postures at hand, the unhelpful, disturbing voice in your head may start again. For instance, let's say that you are teaching a group of three students a series of chaturanga push-ups. Out of nowhere, the self-doubting voice kicks in. As you realize you're in danger of getting lost in self-doubt, ask yourself a question instead, "What are we doing right now?" This immediately brings you back to the present, refocusing your attention outwardly (on what's in front of you —three persons in the push-up position) and you're good to go further. Try it; it's simple; it works.

EPILOGUE

Most people go through life with average tonality skills. Their voices are forgotten. They make accidental noises. Unless they are born with a miracle voice, they never pay much attention to how it sounds, or how others perceive it. They find it difficult to achieve their heart's desire. You are no longer one of those people, are you? You are better than that. You know things now that you didn't know before. "Knowledge is power." You have put the new knowledge into practice and made changes. You have learned to breathe better and take the right stance. You have added volume, created variety in your tone, and much more. I'm proud of you. I'm looking forward to hearing you speak!

ACKNOWLEDGMENTS

First, last, and always, I want to acknowledge the Source who I thank for the Great Design of Everything through which I find meaning in a life which flows somewhere between order and chaos.

Secondly, in a personal way, I am grateful to my Teachers, Family, Friends, Colleagues, Employees, Students, and a few more Persons whose privacy I respect and cannot mention the names of here—each one who has touched my heart and/or my mind in their own way, which defies description.

Thirdly, in still personal but also professional terms, I'd like to thank Jimmy Barkan, Lisa Goodwin, Jim Borsellino, Philip Christodoulou, and the family of teachers at the Barkan Method's home studio in Fort Lauderdale, Florida, who all put up with me during my first steps in hatha yoga and in teaching. Lucas Rockwood of YOGABODY and Absolute Yoga Academy, as well as Harreson Martell and Julie Sceeny, who all have been great partners to work with. Cesar Milan, the Dog Whisperer, from who I learnt some transferable skills (please don't tell my yoga students I said that, but teaching a beginner yoga class or fulfilling your dog's needs for exercise and discipline before affection are rather similar in more ways than one). C.G. Jung, Marie-Louise von Franz, Fyodor Dostoyevsky, Quentin Tarantino, Gordon Ramsay, Eminem, Jerry Seinfeld, Christoph Waltz—your enthusiasm, creative genius, craft, and successes inspire me—thank you. Heidi Ulrich and Andrea Freely of Yoga Moves Nyon, Cherry Wang of YIHE42 Yoga in Beijing, and Christoph Mamat of Sun Yoga Berlin, I am grateful for your support. Izzy ben Natan, Miguel Kirjon, Silvano Stabile (The Game!), Piyanuch Ketnim, Anna Leder, Kiki Bianca, and Marek Koperski have been helpful in making this small book a reality.

ABOUT THE AUTHOR

Tomasz is a writer, educator, yoga teacher (E-RYT 200, YACEP), and yoga course director (RYS 200).

He grew up in a family of artists, including theater actors who he fondly remembers to always have been practicing their lines, their tonalities, and their physical expressions.

Tomasz learnt to teach yoga from Jimmy Barkan in Florida. Jimmy was a film actor before he became one of the most respected teacher trainers in the USA. Tomasz learnt from Jimmy, among other things, how significant voice skills are for any teacher, and how to improve those skills by practice.

Having then quit his professional gambler's career, Tomasz taught over 12,500 hours of yoga classes and teacher trainings in various locations in multi-language and diverse cultural environments. For 7 years, he owned a successful yoga studio and helped other studio owners grow their business. Over the years, Tomasz came to a universal conclusion: the way a yoga teacher sounds makes or breaks their success.

The voice-for-success coaching, which until now you could only get from Tomasz in person during his courses, is available to you in the form of this book.

Tomasz lives in Thailand and teaches in China, Switzerland, Germany, and Poland. Stay tuned for next books from Tomasz on body language, practical teaching skills, and more.

To get updates about the next books:

https://tomaszgoetel.com
tomaszgoe@protonmail.com

THANK YOU!

Just one more thing. You couldn't do me a small favour, could you? Could you go online to Amazon, rate this book, and write a review of it. They will also ask you to tell your friends what you think. If you believe this book is worth a mention, would you take a moment to let people know about it? I'd like for this book to help them like it helped you.

(Even if English is not your first language, please don't be shy to write a few words of a review.)

Thank you, dear Reader, for trusting me with your time. May our paths cross soon, I'd love to hear how you sound.

www.ingramcontent.com/pod-product-compliance
Lightning Source LLC
Chambersburg PA
CBHW050408290526
45786CB00003B/1181